Let's See What's Inside Of Me!!

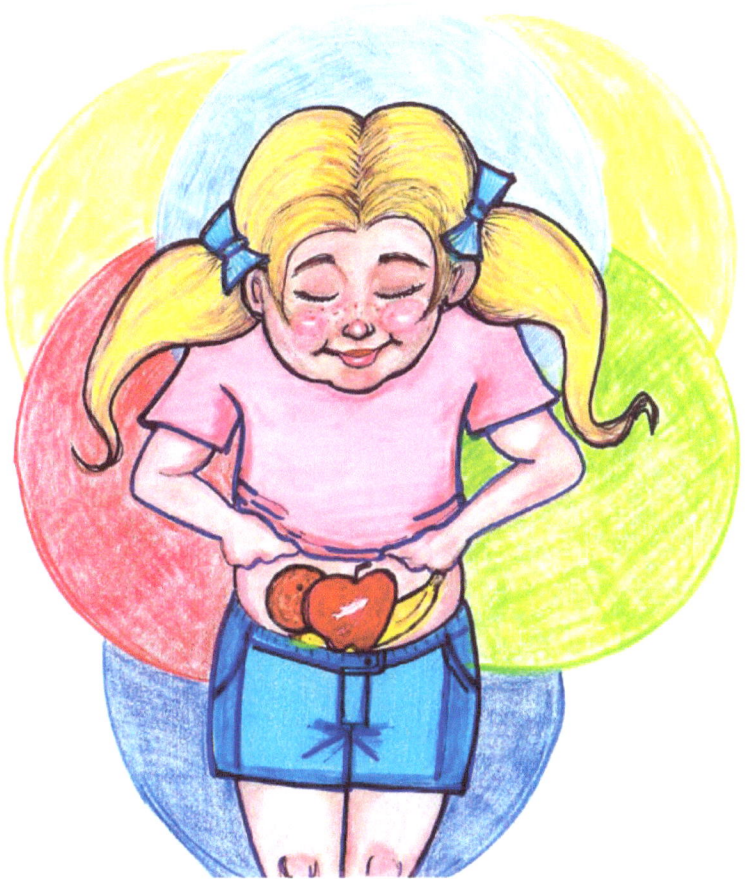

WLL Enterprises, Inc.
An Accredited Business with the Better Business Bureau
P.O. Box 5273, Carson, CA. 90749 USA
www.wllenterprisesinc.org

Copyright 2017, Leslie Wilkes, All Rights Reserved
Book: Let's See What's Inside of Me
Date Published: 10/2017 /Edition 1 Trade Paperback
ISBN: 978-0-692-96945-8

This book was published in Compton, California
United States of America

A Publisher Trademark Title Page

LET'S SEE WHAT'S INSIDE OF ME

100% of the proceeds from the sale of this book will go to
WLL Enterprises Inc.
WLL Enterprises Inc. is a Non-Profit Organization dedicated
to fighting Childhood Obesity.

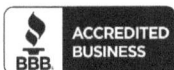

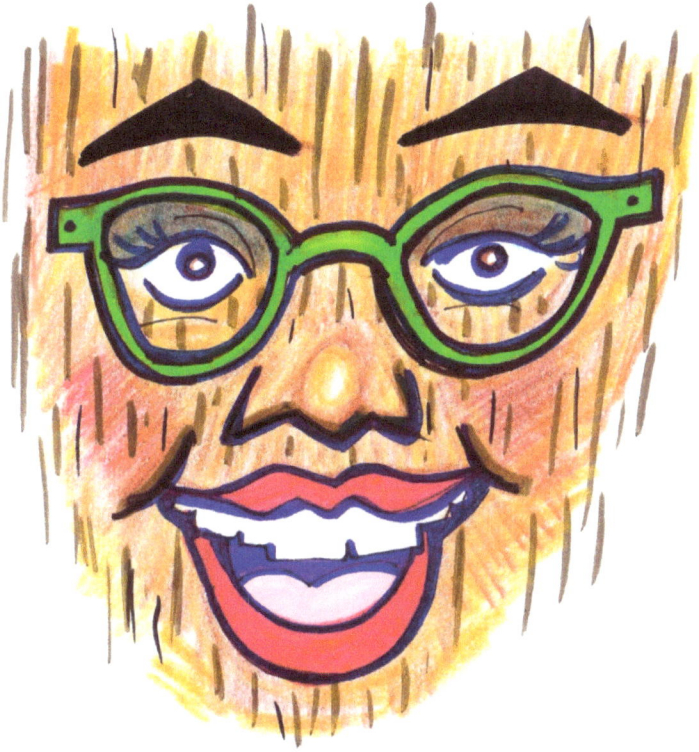

Good Morning class, welcome to your first day of school.

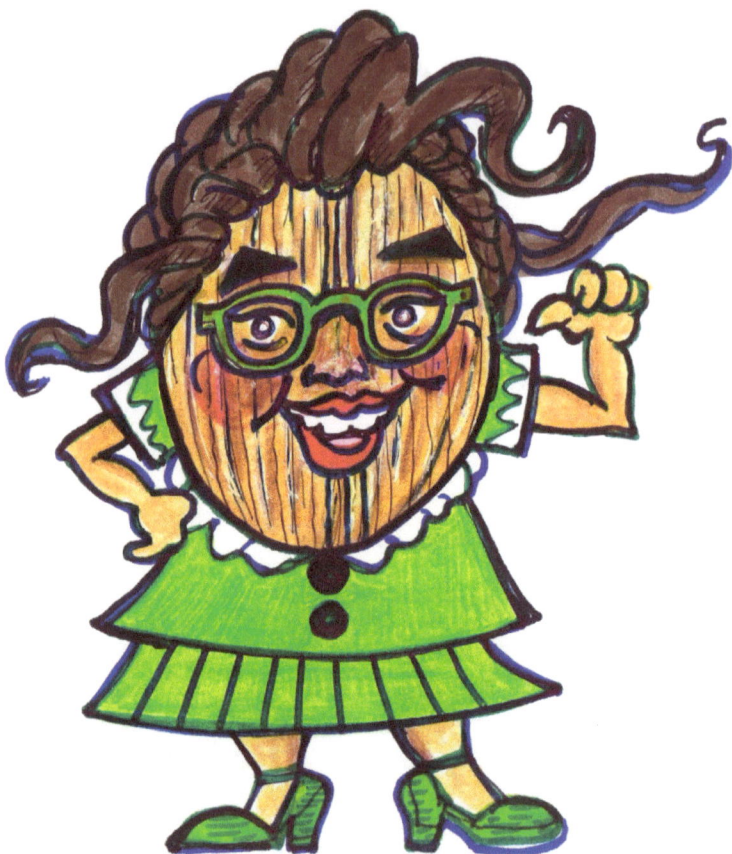

My name is Mrs. Walnut and I'm a nut, I have vitamin E in me. I want each one of you to come up and tell the class who you are.

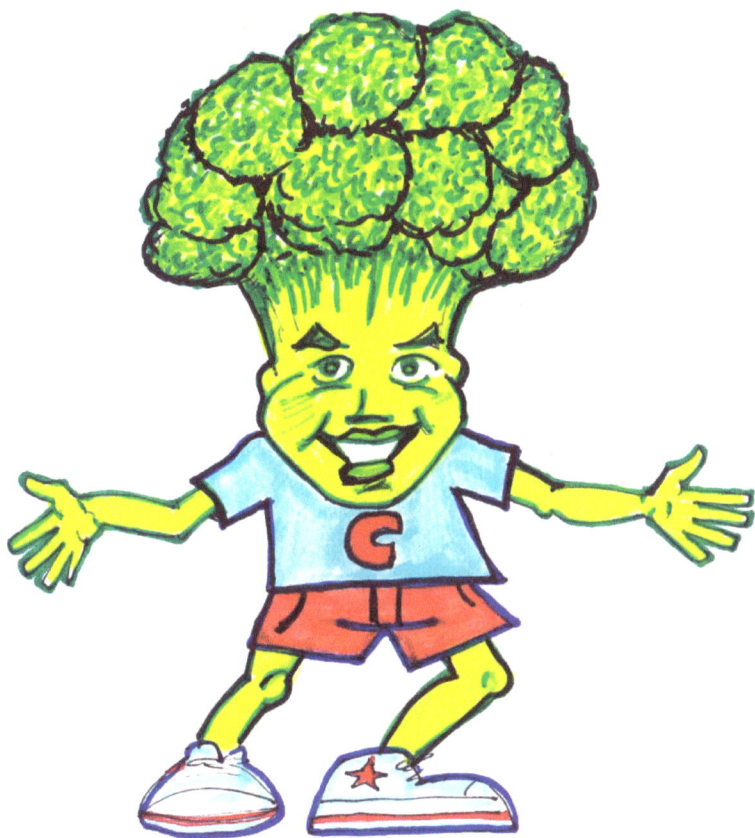

My name is Broccoli and I'm a vegetable, I can be white, orange, purple and green. I have vitamin C in me.

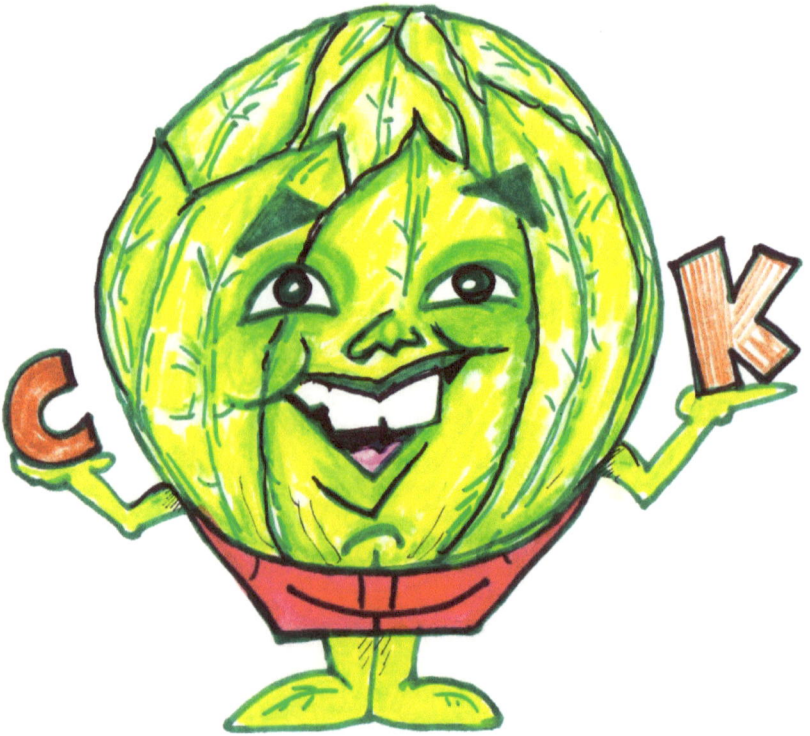

My name is Cabbage and I'm a vegetable, I can be green or purple. I have vitamin C and K in me.

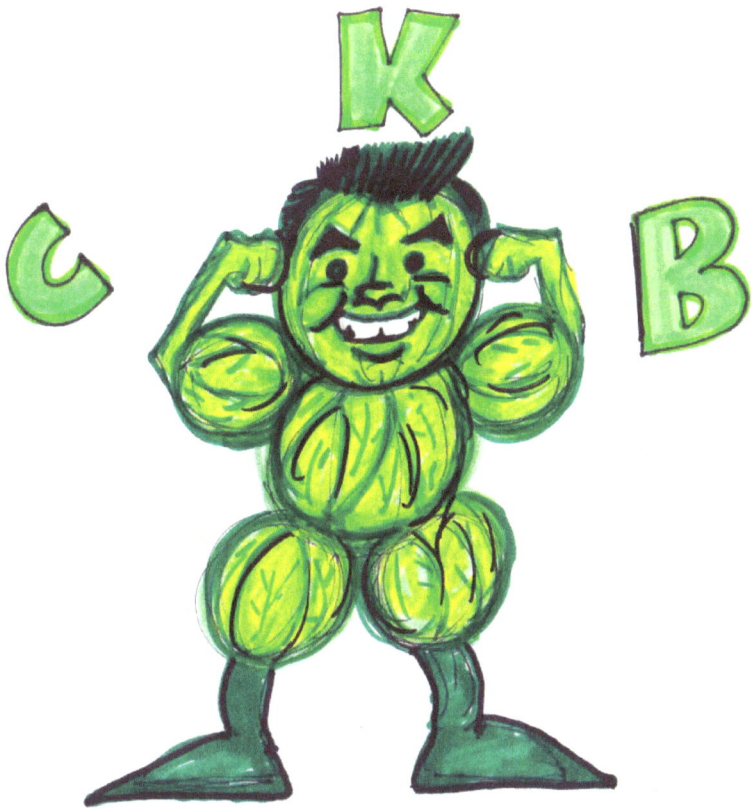

My name is Brussel Sprout and I'm a vegetable, I am green and I have vitamins C, K and B in me.

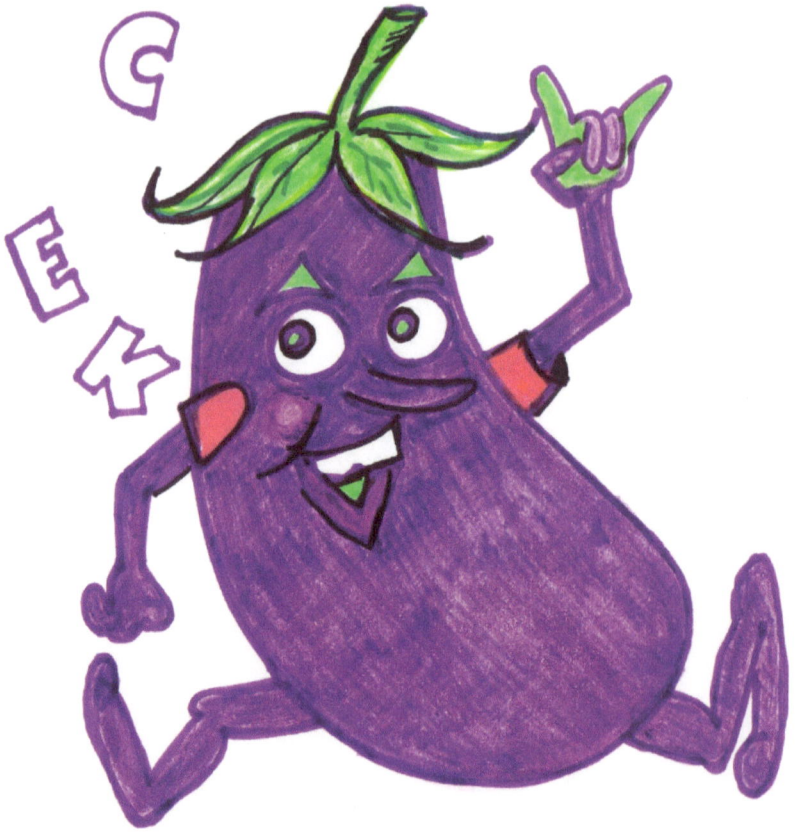

My name is Eggplant and I am purple and I'm a fruit, I have vitamins C, E and K in me.

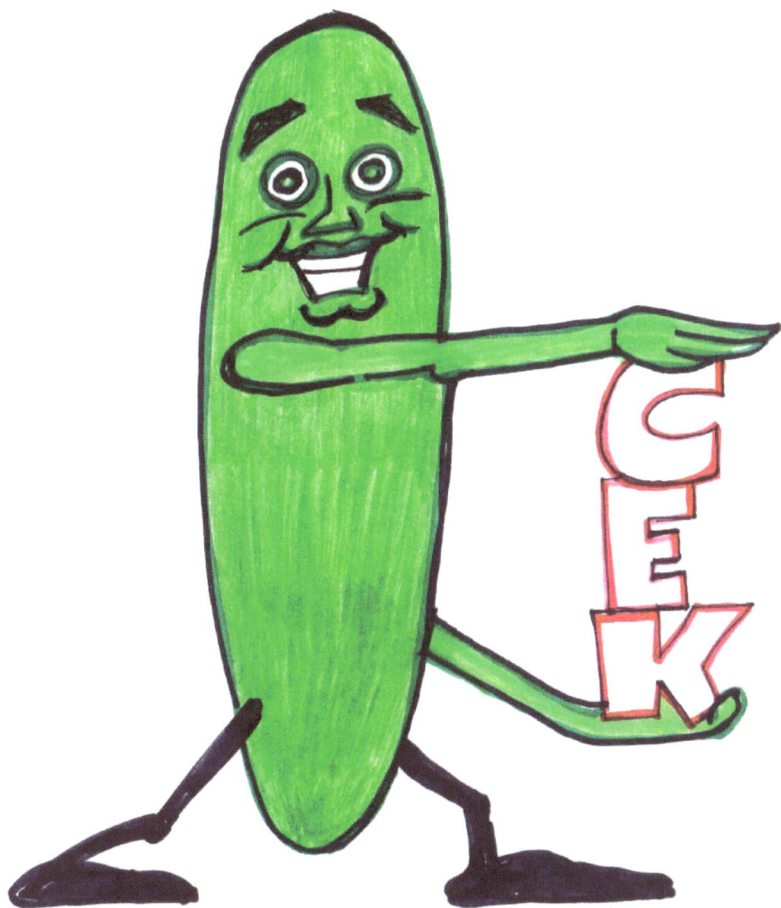

My name is Cucumber and technically I'm a fruit, I am green and I have vitamins C, E and K in me.

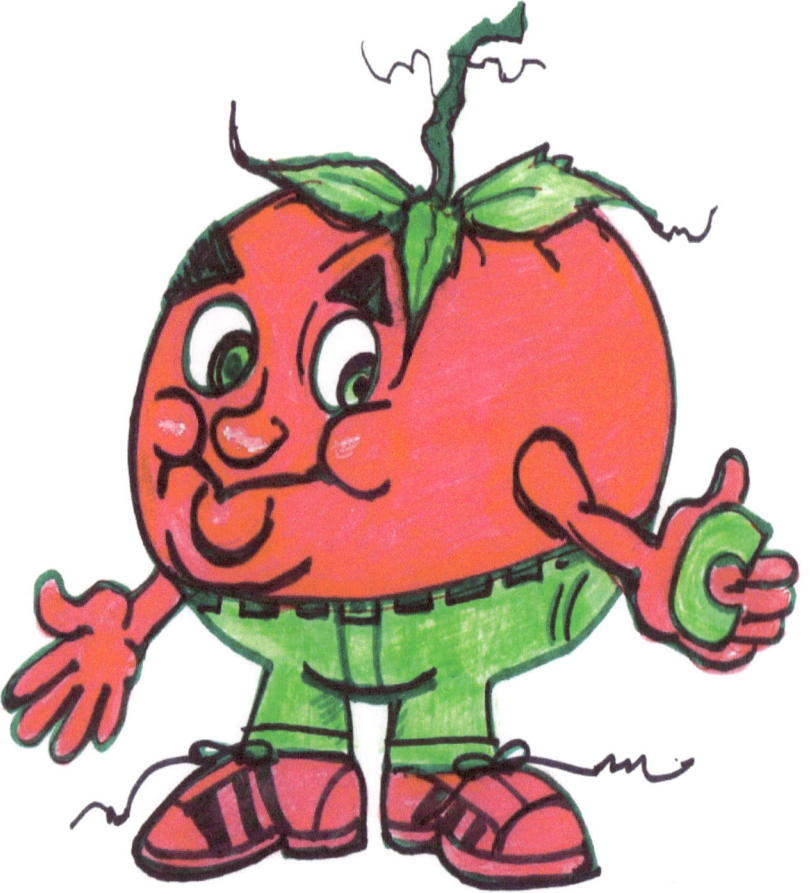

My name is Tomato and I am a fruit,
and I have vitamin C in me.

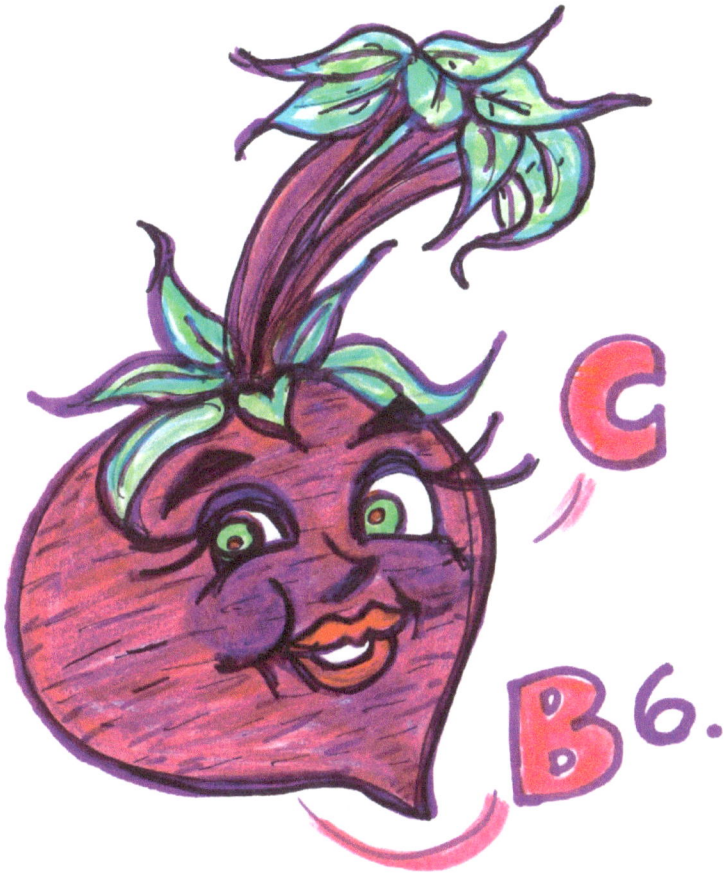

My name is Beet and I'm a vegetable,
I'm red and I have vitamin C and B6.

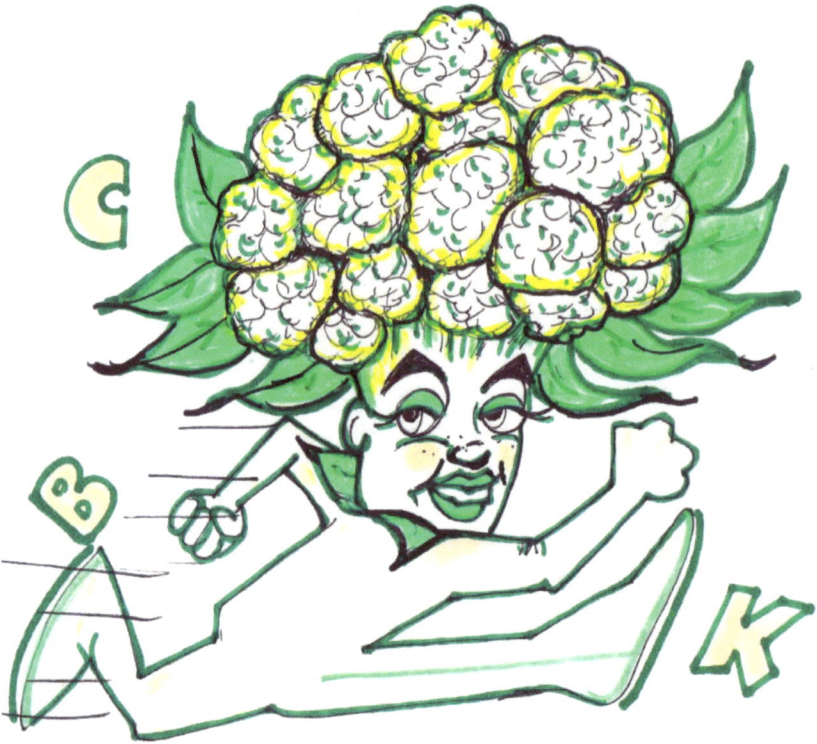

My name is Cauliflower and I'm a vegetable, I can be white, orange, green or purple. I have vitamins C, B and K in me.

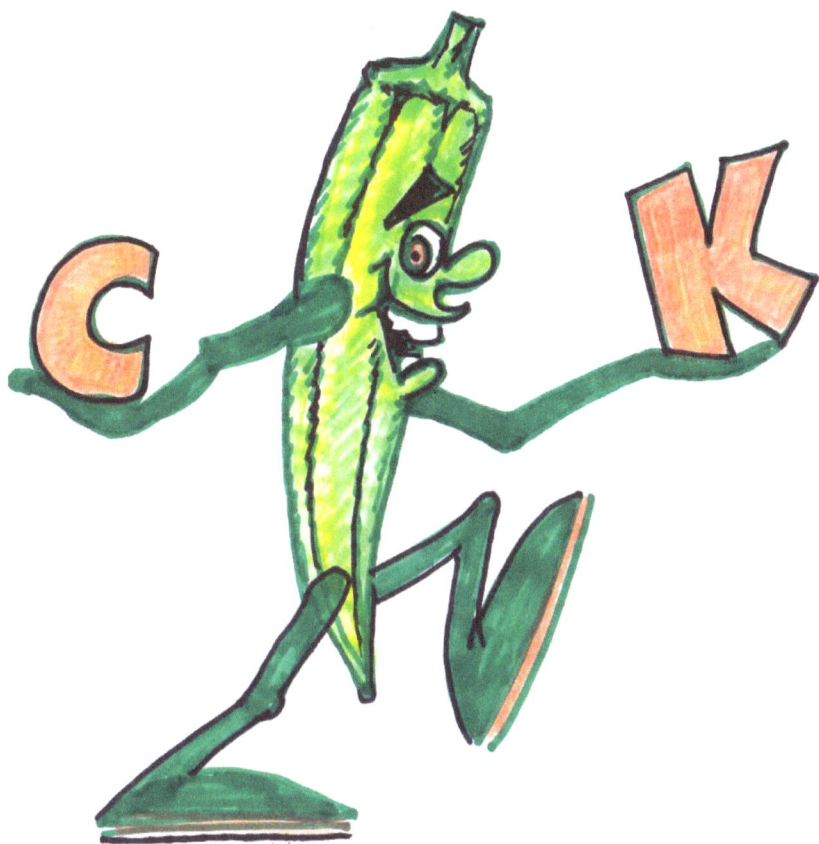

My name is Okra and I'm a vegetable,
I have vitamins C and K in me.

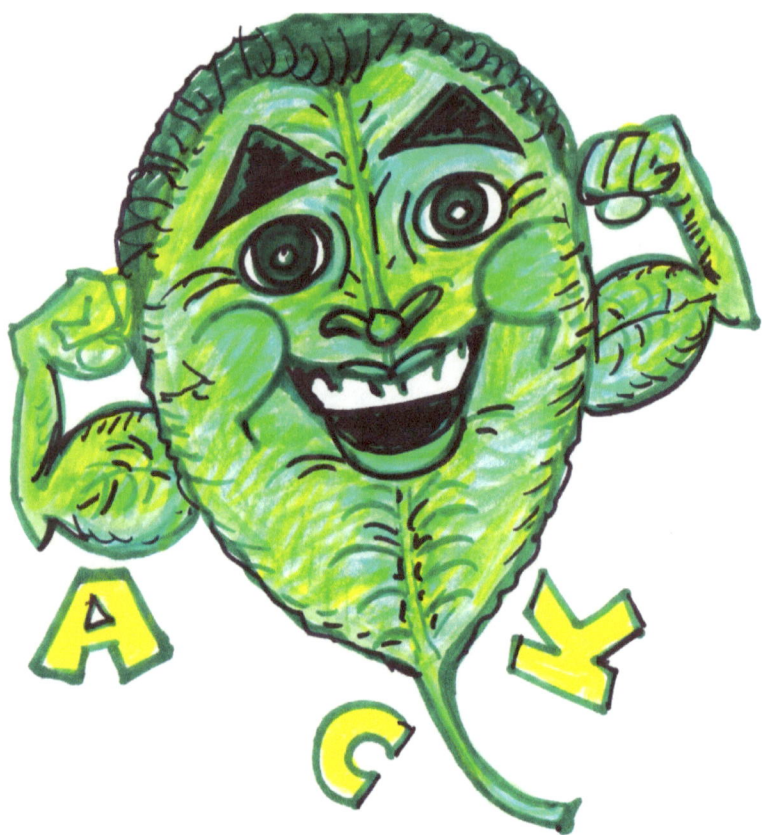

My name is Spinach and I'm a vegetable, I have vitamins A, C and K in me.

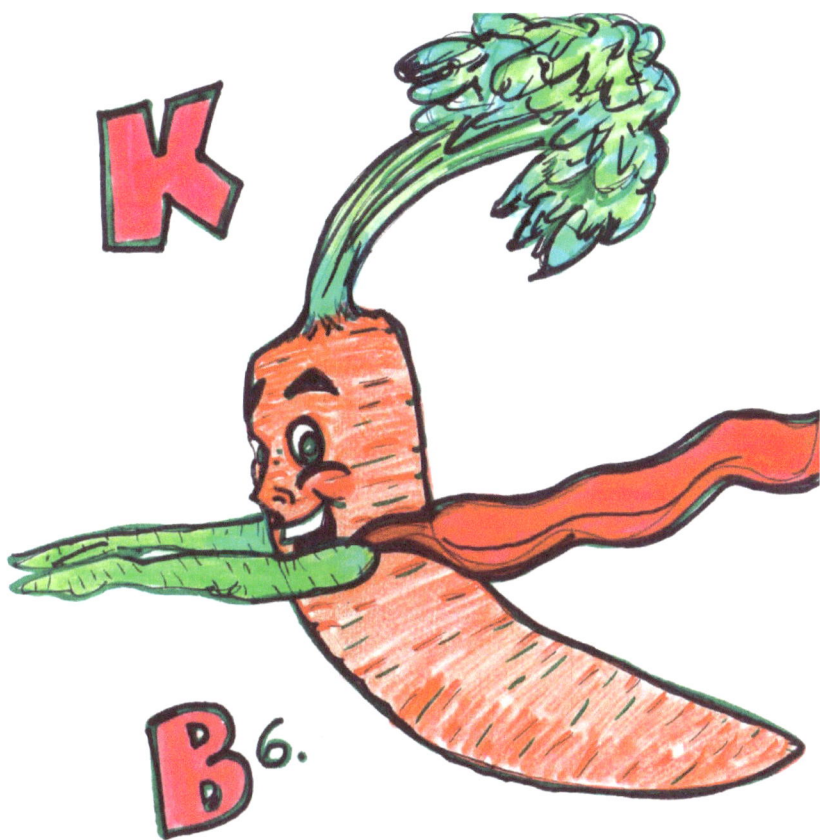

My name is Carrot and I'm a vegetable, I can be orange, black, purple, white, red and yellow. I have vitamins K and B6 in me.

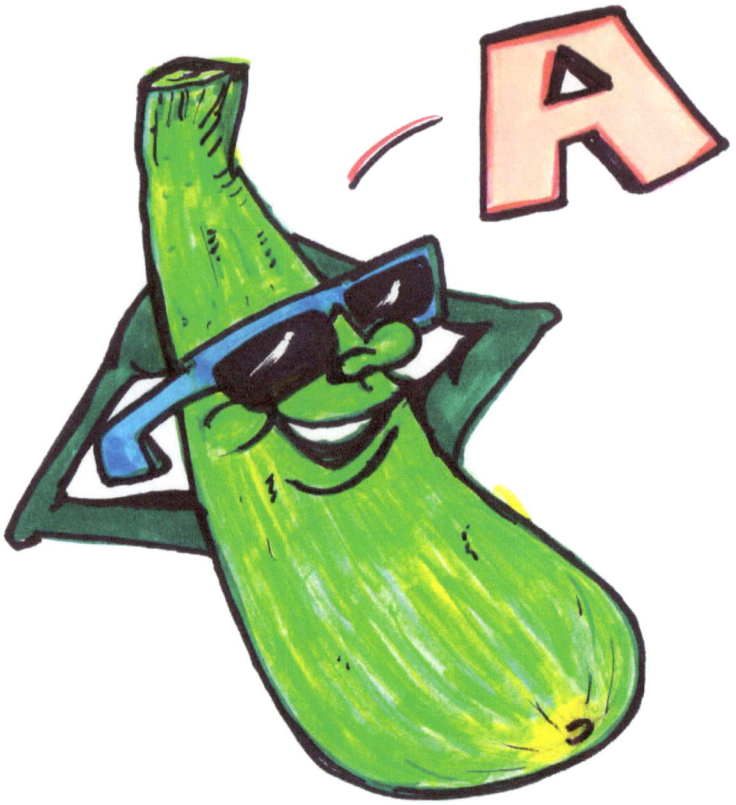

My name is Zucchini and I'm a fruit, I have vitamin A in me.

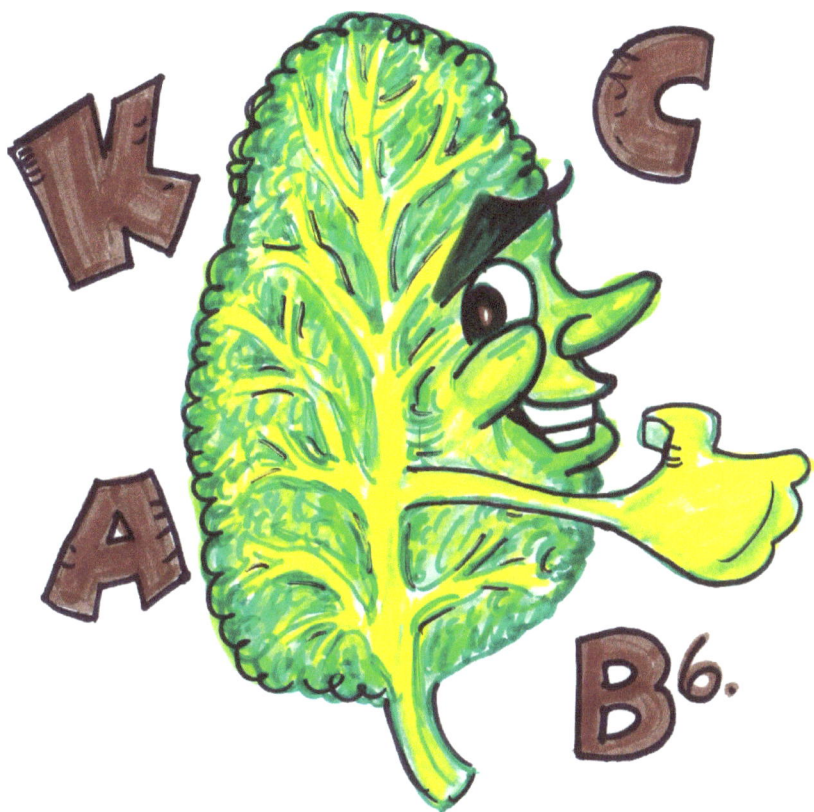

My name is Kale and I'm a vegetable, I have vitamins K, A, C and B6.

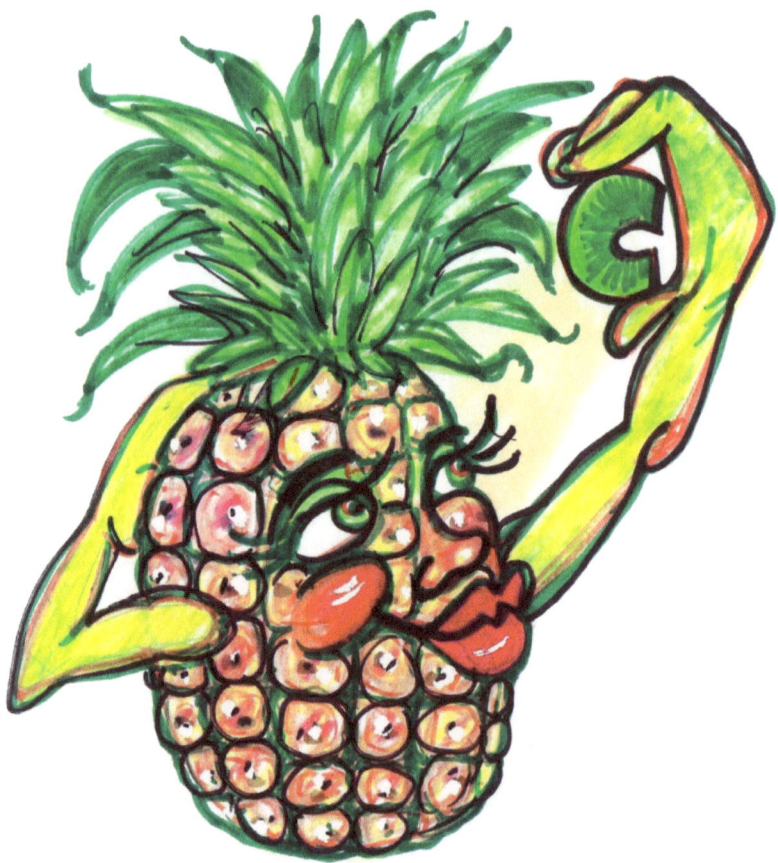

My name is Pineapple and I'm a fruit, I have vitamin C in me.

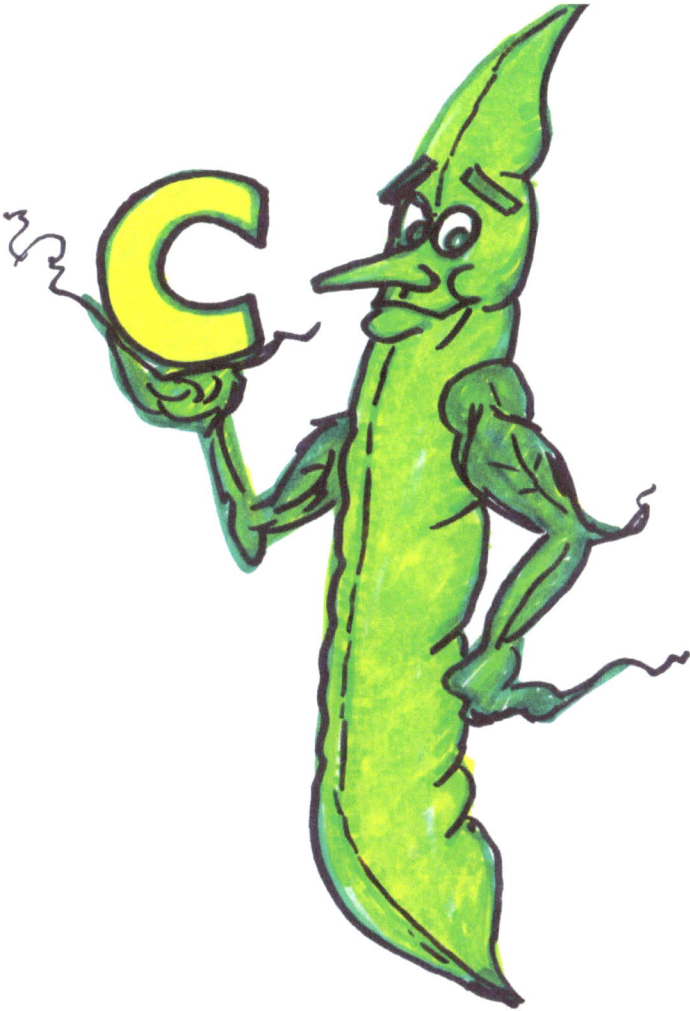

My name is Green Bean and I'm
technically a fruit, I have vitamins C
and K in me.

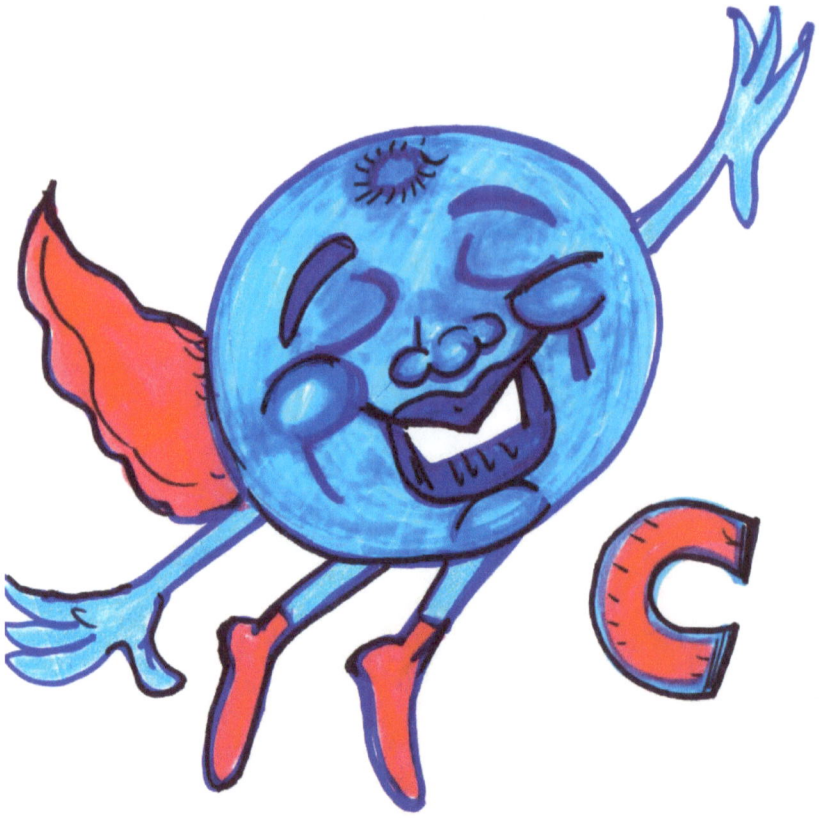

My name is Blueberry and I'm a fruit, I have vitamin C in me.

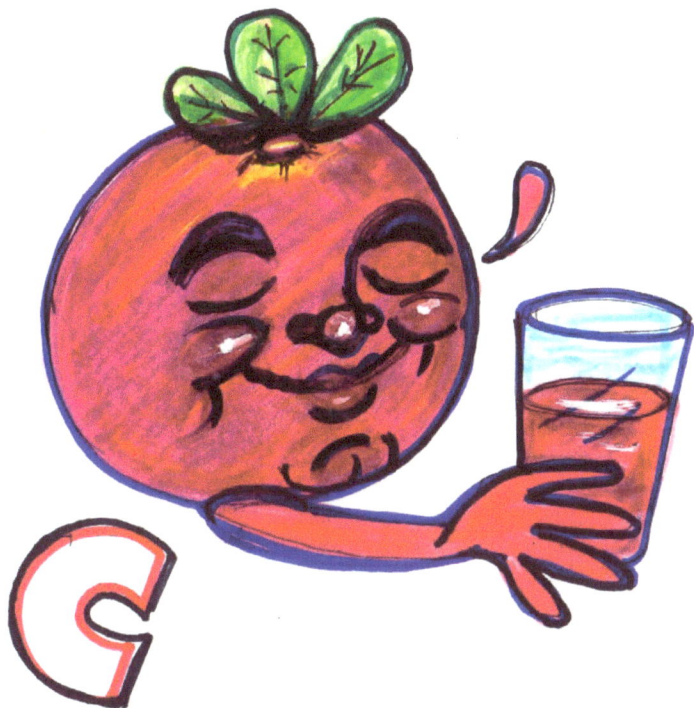

My name is Cranberry and I'm a fruit, I have vitamin C in me.

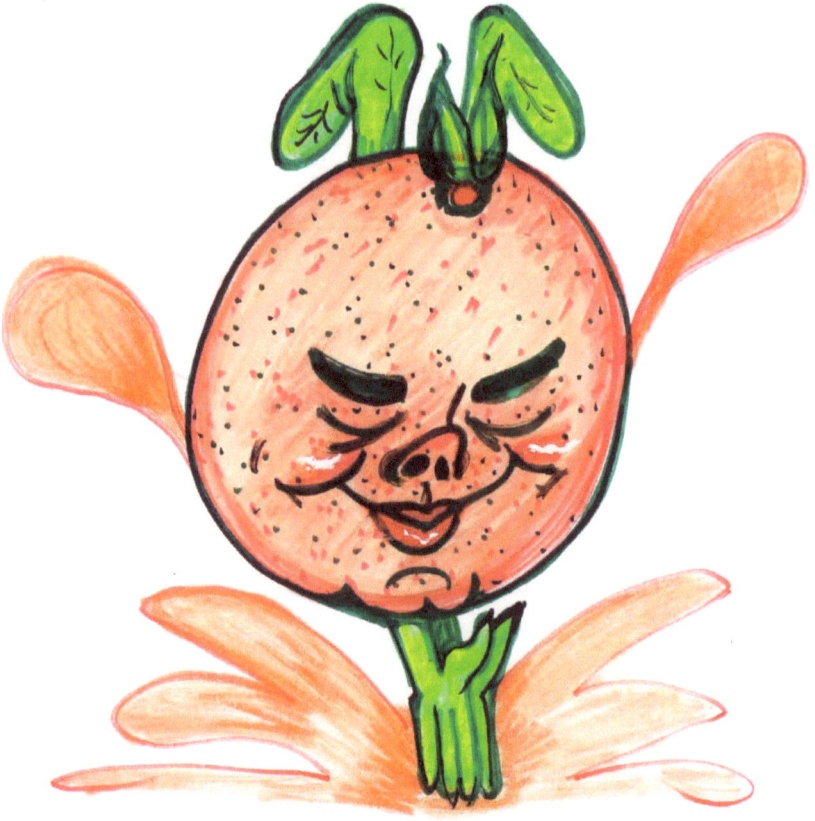

My name is Orange and I'm a fruit, I
have vitamin C in me.

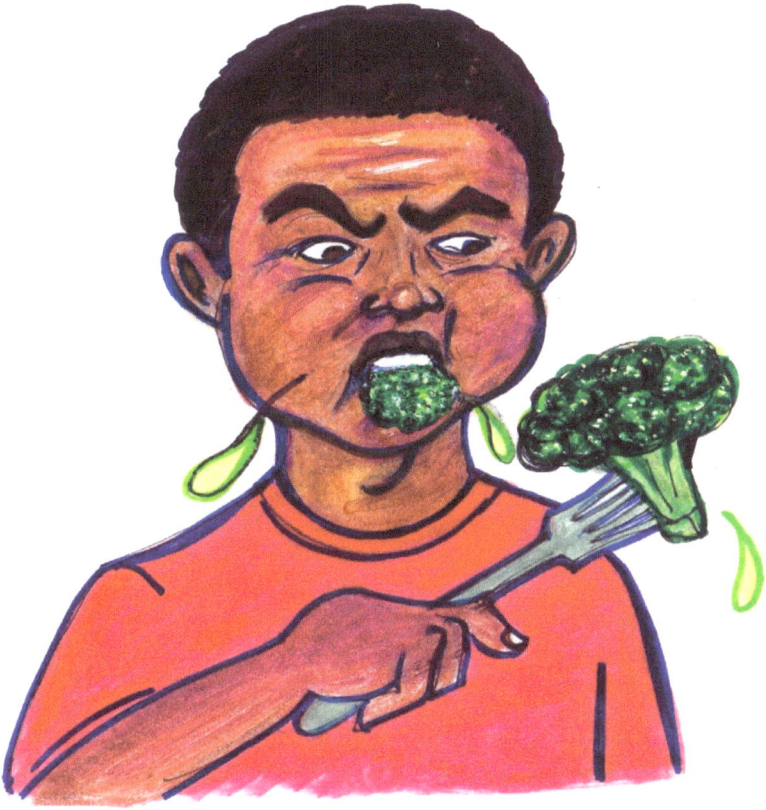

Eating fruits and vegetables is not popular among our youth I know.

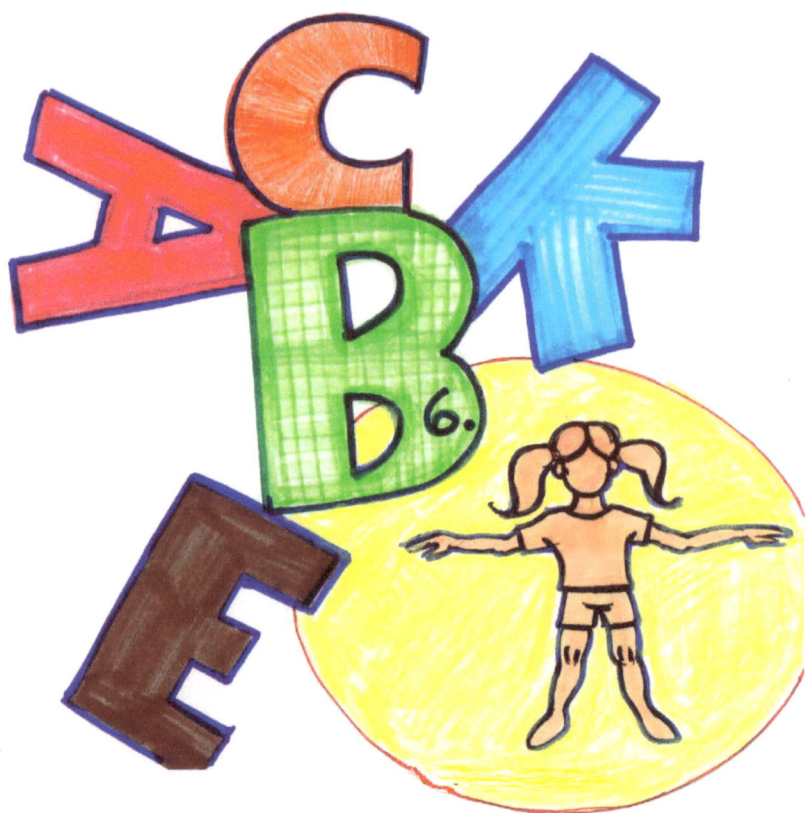

Vitamins play an important part in
your body development.

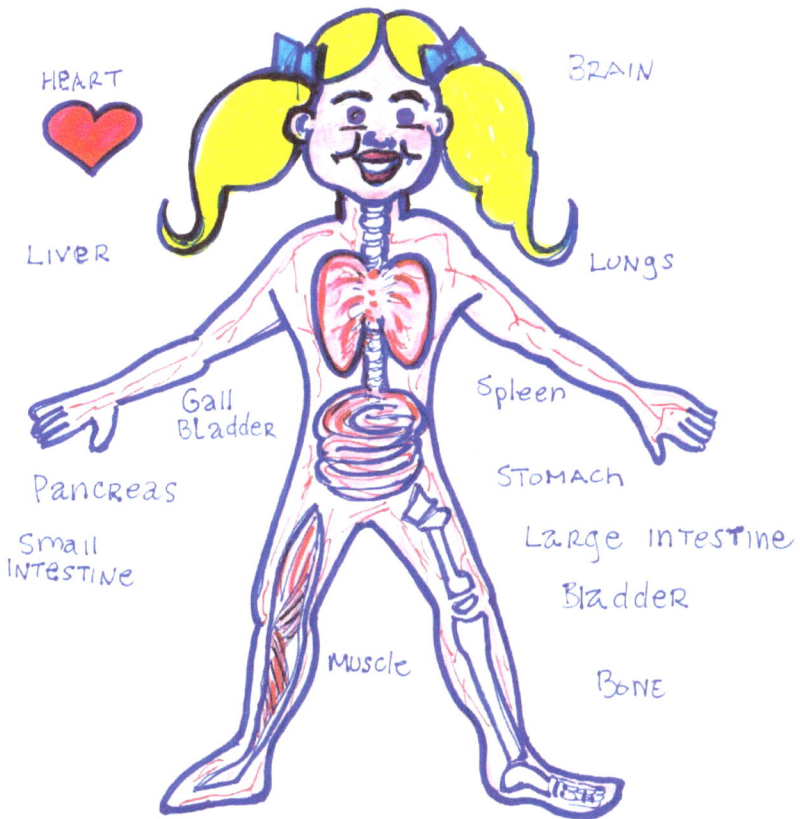

HEART

BRAIN

LIVER

LUNGS

Gall Bladder

Spleen

Pancreas

STOMACH

Small INTESTINE

LARGE INTESTINE

Bladder

Muscle

BONE

With all of us together we help in your development and growth, we also help keep your immune system healthy.

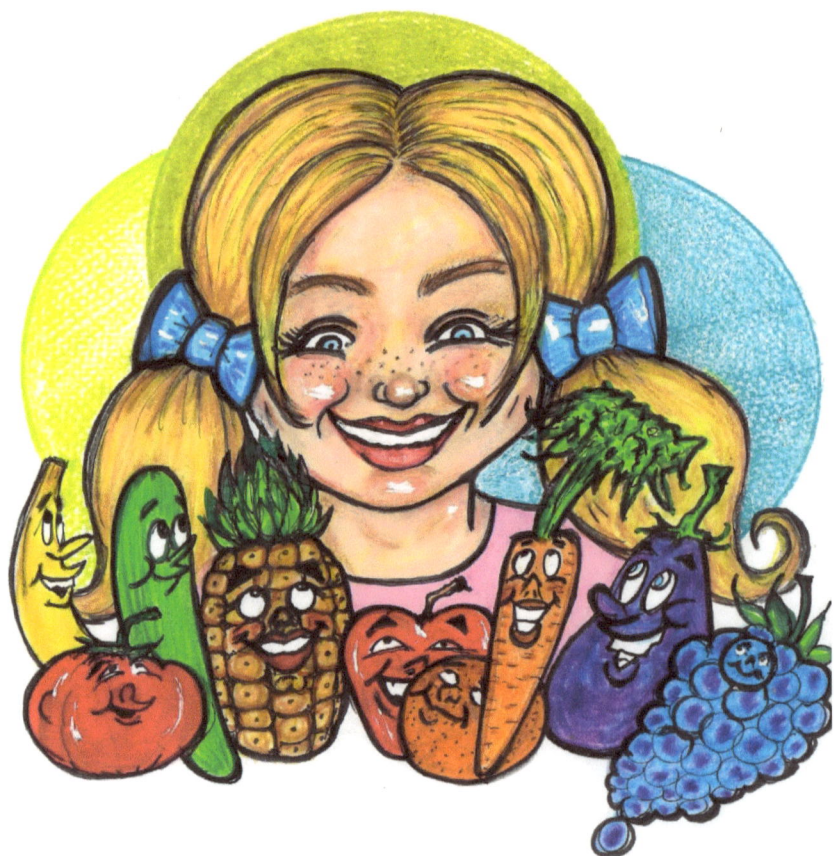

Keeping us in you, will help you live a happy healthy life...

www.ingramcontent.com/pod-product-compliance
Lightning Source LLC
Chambersburg PA
CBHW041215270326
41930CB00001B/36